HOW TO MEND
A BROKEN HEART

T0167784

ZIELLA BRYARS

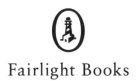

Fairlight Books

First published by Fairlight Books 2021

Fairlight Books
Summertown Pavilion, 18–24 Middle Way, Oxford, OX2 7LG

A CIP catalogue record for this book is available from the British Library.

1 2 3 4 5 6 7 8 9 10

ISBN 978-1-912054-32-9

www.fairlightbooks.com

Printed and bound in Great Britain

Cover designed by Amanda Weiss

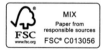

CONTENTS

CHAPTER ONE

Broken-Hearted

Hello, my broken-hearted friend. I'm so sorry this has happened. Who knew something that sounded as sweet and enticing as romance could also punch so hard?

How much more validating it would be if a broken heart were called by some impressive medical name that you could announce with great seriousness to all your friends. 'Did you hear Amy has *heartbreak*?! My God, what bad luck to catch it right at the end of winter.' You could take sick leave, your symptoms would be respected and you wouldn't think you were going mad when you didn't bounce back as quickly as you'd like. You would have contracted heartbreak and everyone would take it as seriously as you.

The reality of how bad heartbreak can be first hit me when, years ago, I came down with a particularly bad case of the broken hearts. I have in fact been heartbroken many a time, but this was the break-up that knocked me the hardest. I was at that dangerous meeting point of being both completely loved up and utterly unprepared. And almost worse than the shock was how embarrassed I felt. It had been a kind of undefined relationship without a proper name. Sometimes on, sometimes off. Sometimes clear and sometimes not. I felt like I wasn't entitled to feel as bad as I did – and yet it was as if I had been punched in the gut.

That was when, without warning, I was suddenly unable to eat. The smell of food, the idea of it, everything to do with eating made me nauseous. The experience was like having gastric flu, but I wasn't sick in the traditional sense: I was heartbroken. I am not someone who ever misses a meal. I do not forget to have lunch because I'm too busy. I love food, I love cooking, I love thinking about food and thinking about cooking. To be so in shock and so sad that my stomach hurt was like nothing I had ever experienced before. For someone who had never felt a tie between her body and her heart, it was a fascinating – if upsetting – realisation. My broken heart had, temporarily, broken me.

Luckily for me I had a very close and incredibly clever friend to help me through it. A neuroscientist, no less. My wise, kind, brilliant friend Sarah, who spends her days scanning brains while the rest of us send emails, was, by wonderful chance, the person by my side at that sad and confusing moment. Her way of talking about heartache came from a completely different place to the advice I was used to. I didn't want to eat? she asked. Well, that made sense. In periods of stress the HPA axis is activated, resulting in higher levels of the stress hormone cortisol and increased autonomic arousal, and these changes can impact the digestive system. Didn't I know that? No. I did not. My tips on heartbreak came from magazines. I thought I was meant to get a haircut.

Her way of looking at the world gave me hope and guidance in those awful first few weeks. Her scientific approach to life, rooted in fact, was so refreshing and calm. So much so that I started trying to log all the useful little nuggets of information she would give me. I saved articles she sent me; I wrote down things she said in notes on my phone; I even started to seek out scientific studies on my own, not only for my future dumped self but for the many coffees, movie nights and meals ahead I knew I would have with fellow heartbroken friends.

The more articles I read and the more I talked to Sarah, the more reassurance I felt. Every time she started a sentence with 'Did you know that research shows…', I felt a tiny bit saner. There was such relief in hearing that the sensations I was experiencing were not down to madness or weakness; they were not about me being melodramatic or silly or naive. Each fact and each study I read made me realise that I wasn't personally having some overly dramatic reaction or breaking down – this was my brain and my body recovering from a real, documented and scientifically recognised impact. In fact, in a way, the process I was going through was what made me, along with every other human on the planet, so brilliant, rather than making us weak. I had a Chemistry teacher once who told our class that when he got into debates with his more poetic friends, they would become frustrated about how analytically he saw the world, how scientists dissected everything and didn't look at something like a beautiful rose and just say 'Wow, that's so stunning and magical.' 'But don't you see,' he said to his class full of cynical teenagers, 'the atoms and molecules that make up that rose, the pigment that makes it red and not pink, the chance of it blooming or existing at all in the miniscule strip of liveable atmosphere that skirts the outside of our planet

are what make it so much more mind-blowing to look at.'
For once I think our entire class was listening. I remember
feeling in that moment that he probably saw more magic in
a bunch of flowers than the rest of us.

Now, I am as guilty as the next person of reading trashy
magazines and crying along to break-up songs – I went
through a country music phase for this very reason – but
sometimes we need a little more than a haircut or a playlist
to help us through an experience like this. Sometimes we
need something more solid to hold on to. Understanding
what was happening inside my body and mind not only
helped me to be kinder to myself but also steered me towards
some helpful coping strategies. Our instincts are not always
the best during this time, so a little help from the world of
science can be a useful tool.

Do you want to know what is extra unfair about being
heartbroken? Our IQ actually decreases. Our logic and
reasoning are impaired and our judgement is altered. I know
– what a treat. Like we haven't got enough to deal with right
now. Studies on how emotions affect logical reasoning show
that the state we are in when we are heartbroken has a clear

effect on our performance in even relatively simple tasks.[1] Our competence actually goes down. We are also more likely to draw illogical conclusions as our emotions continue to have an impact on our reasoning[2] and, on top of this, studies on negative emotional states and their influence on logic show that any beliefs we have going into a task or scenario are more likely than usual to outweigh our normal powers of deduction.[3] A heartbroken person is a biased, illogical muddle – scientifically speaking. If ever I needed my brain to be working at full capacity, it was in those first few post-break-up weeks. I could have done with some *increased* reasoning, thank you very much, but apparently that is not the way it goes. Not only are we navigating painful new terrain, but we are actually less clever as we do so.

This may not be the most positive heartbreak fact to start off with, but, honestly, isn't it better to know? Don't we want to understand what's going on inside our confused minds right now? To know that as we struggle more than usual in this difficult time, there is a reason for it. A scientific, studied-in-labs reason. We don't have to feel frustrated or think we are losing our minds. We don't have to feel crazy or silly on

[1] Jung, N. et al. 'How emotions affect logical reasoning: Evidence from experiments with mood-manipulated participants, spider phobics, and people with exam anxiety', *Frontiers in Psychology*, 5 (2014), 570. doi:10.3389/fpsyg.2014.00570

[2] Blanchette, I. and Richards, A. 'Reasoning about emotional and neutral materials: Is logic affected by emotion?', *Psychological Science*, 15(11) (2004), 745–52. doi:10.1111/j.0956-7976.2004.00751

[3] Goel, V. and Vartanian, O. 'Negative emotions can attenuate the influence of beliefs on logical reasoning', *Cognition and Emotion*, 25(1) (2011), 121–31. doi:10.1080/02699931003593942

top of feeling sad. We can breathe a sigh of relief and know that this is happening to everyone's brain in this state. This is normal, this is measurable, this even shows up on an MRI scan. If we can understand what is going on inside us as we process our broken hearts, we have a much greater chance of coping with the side effects and, ultimately, recovering.

Although I didn't end up taking a scientific path in my career, instead writing things like rom-coms rather than groundbreaking research papers, I think perhaps my Chemistry teacher planted a little seed in my mind that is best nurtured by data and statistics. The calm reassurance I feel on reading studies about heartbreak definitely seems to come from an inner science geek I didn't realise I had. There is such relief in knowing that heartbreak happens on a neurophysiological level – that it is real and that it affects us to a measurable degree. The clever neuroscientists out there (my best friend among them) who study and research the inner workings of our brains not only have the science to explain what is happening to us but can actually help us in this difficult time. I know Sarah helped me. I also know that without our conversations I would have had more questionable haircuts, done more drunk-dialling and made many more impulse purchases. Understanding the impact that a break-up can have on our bodies and minds can help us figure out what we are going through and how to recover from it. For me, my conversations with Sarah and my new love of heartbreak science not only restored my ravenous (and sometimes commented-on) appetite but also helped me to come out the other side and feel like myself again.

CHAPTER TWO

What Just Happened?

If you're anything like me, you may be spending a lot of time right now staring at the ceiling and asking: 'What the bleeping bleep is going on?' This is not the destination we were aiming for. We didn't head out on that first date, full of nerves and hope and ever-so-slightly rehearsed anecdotes, just to end up weepy and heartbroken. What a strange, masochistic strategy that would be. It is surreal to look around and wonder where everything we had ten minutes ago has suddenly gone.

The feeling of loss that accompanies heartbreak can be hard to comprehend. It feels like someone has died, but the person we have lost is still very much alive. They're walking around town, popping into the bank or buying a muffin, while we feel as if they have evaporated. Our imaginations are powerful things – I know that when I was feeling at my worst, mascara-stained and stuck on the sofa, my brain would always picture my heartbreaker jogging down the beach or high-fiving someone at the gym. It is so strange to think that, while we are feeling this dreadful, they are still alive and out in the world, living out some kind of rom-com-style musical montage. That elusive definition of what exactly heartbreak is and what sort of process we are meant to be going through was something I asked Sarah about on repeat, and probably every other friend I talked to at that time as well. Am I in mourning? Am I in shock? How can I hope to recover if I don't quite understand what this state really is?

What Is Heartbreak?

Feeling so sad and confused was something I could only really compare to grief. But that felt a little melodramatic. No one had actually died. I wasn't sure it was fair, even in the secret deepest depths of my mind, to think about heartbreak in that way. I didn't want to behave like a deluded teenager, throwing herself down on the bed and shouting that her life was over – but if I was honest, it did feel a little like my life was over, or at least as if part of it was. Science suggests, though, that I was not being insensitive in comparing my distress to something as serious as grief. When we are heartbroken, we *are* in a state of grief. This is not just a label we use metaphorically; studies actually show that the loss of a romantic relationship elicits the same reaction in the brain as a bereavement.[4]

Mourning for Beginners

Thinking of heartbreak as a form of grief can help us understand the confused, scrambled sensations that often follow a break-up. Let's for a moment consider the state our brain is in when we lose someone we love. MRI scans of bereaved participants have shown that a particular area of the brain is activated when we experience grief: the posterior cingulate cortex, to be precise.[5] In her review on romantic breakup distress, Dr Tiffany M. Field reveals that MRI scans of participants experiencing heartbreak actually show the same regional brain activity as people experiencing a bereavement.[6] When we are heartbroken we really are in mourning, and the brain responds to the loss of

4Field, T. M. 'Romantic breakup distress, betrayal and heartbreak: A review', *International Journal of Behavioral Research and Psychology*, 5(2) (2017), 217–25 (220). doi: http://dx.doi.org/10.19070/2332-3000-1700038

5Gündel, H., O'Connor, M.-F., Littrell, L., Fort, C. and Lane R. D. 'Functional neuroanatomy of grief: An FMRI study', *American Journal of Psychiatry*, 160(11) (2003), 1946–53. doi:10.1176/appi.ajp.160.11.1946

6Najib, A., Lorberbaum, J. P., Kose, S., Bohning, D. E. and George, M. S. 'Regional brain activity in women grieving a romantic relationship breakup', *American Journal of Psychiatry*, 161(12) (2004), 2245–56. doi:10.1176/appi.ajp.161.12.2245

a relationship in the same way that it does to the death of a loved one. The sensations of shock and, in some cases, denial that we can experience after a break-up are not dissimilar to those generated by grief. In light of this similarity, the confused, shocked, lost feeling we have at first when we are heartbroken does not seem so strange.

In the early days of a broken heart you are likely to feel pretty unsettled. Your brain is scrambled; you are searching for what is true and what is false. You are likely to be replaying a lot of scenes in your head in flashes and broken sequences, like a badly cut music video. For me, it is what I call my David Lynch phase, in which – as anyone who has seen his movies will know – the floor is not always the floor, you might walk through a front door and end up on the roof, and sometimes your neighbour turns into a doorknob (real David Lynch storyline). Your brain's attempt to reconcile what it thought was real with what is actually happening can be an overwhelming experience. I use the David Lynch example not to be poetic but because this state really does feel cinematic somehow. You can feel the camera swerve around you as you try to catch your breath and figure out where you now stand. Yes, the person we have lost may in this case still be alive – they may even be happily jogging down a beach – but this doesn't mean we are not reeling from the death of the relationship.

When our mind experiences the kind of impact that bereavement generates, the first thing it does is try to protect us. The commonly referred to 'stages of grief', first introduced by Elisabeth Kübler-Ross in her book *On Death and Dying*,[7] typically begin with the state of denial or shock, and studies in the area of heartbreak recognise that the loss of a relationship triggers the same bereavement-like symptoms.[8] Struggling to comprehend this reality is therefore not an unusual reaction. Our brain wants to protect us and at first that protection can come in the form of denial. Denial sounds so negative – like we are cowardly for not facing up to what is right in front of us – but it is in fact a helpful, protective tool. Denial is a device that the brain engages to prevent greater trauma, initially preventing our minds from processing the distressing reality we are presented with and helping to give us time to absorb everything at a slower rate. Our brain is wired to protect us from information that could cause us harm. It can block even the most basic 'truths' if this information could be too distressing.

[7] Kübler-Ross, E. *On Death and Dying*. Oxford: Routledge, 1969.
[8] Field, T. 'Romantic breakups, heartbreak and bereavement', *Psychology*, 2(4) (2011), 382–87. doi:10.4236/psych.2011.24060

Researchers at Bar-Ilan University in Israel exploring the brain's use of denial have shown that when the brain is presented with information about our own mortality it shields us from it. To prevent us from having an existential crisis, it processes the concept of mortality as something that can only happen to other people. It turns a fact we know logically to be true into something else in order to keep us alive and prevent our basic sense of purpose from collapsing.[9] In the Bar-Ilan University study, when participants were presented with images of other people alongside the concept of death, the brain accepted that combination – but when an image of themselves was presented alongside these ideas, the brain shut down the possibility of this connection. It would accept the death of others but not of the self.

I love this kind of study. It is scientifically fascinating while also being mildly comical. I can picture a cartoon brain sticking its fingers in its ears and singing 'La-la-la-la!' And mortality isn't the only thing our brains are good at ignoring: I know there were times early on in my worst ever heartbreak when I would pretty much do the same thing and just think: 'Nope! Not happening!' It is understandable and, in fact, helpful that we are in denial at first. It is an early reaction to grief and forms part of the bereavement-like state we are in. It is the clever

[9]Dor-Ziderman, Y., Lutz, A. and Goldstein, A. 'Prediction-based neural mechanisms for shielding the self from existential threat', *NeuroImage*, 202 (2019), 116080. doi:10.1016/j.neuroimage.2019.116080

strategy our brains use in order to form a protective, murky fog around us. It may not feel fun to exist within this fog, but it is not something to fight against, and we don't need to feel silly for experiencing this. We are not confused because we are flawed – we are confused because our minds are brilliant and protective.

It is not only this state of denial that heartbreak and grief share. Bereavement-like symptoms have been shown to follow most types of romantic loss[10] – from the physical impacts that are explored in the next chapter to intrusive thoughts, depression, sleep disturbances and even something called broken-heart syndrome. This is a rare situation where the emotional impact of loss can actually trigger a heart attack: a very specific kind of heart attack that, on examination of the person after the episode, shows no clogged arteries and no cardiac enzymes released from damaged heart muscles. This heart attack is not caused by a biological trigger but is brought on by the emotional shock induced by intense grief.[11] As far as our heartbreak goes we do not need to worry – we are extremely unlikely to be in this danger zone, as the level of shock created would have to be very high from a break-up as opposed to the sudden,

[10]Davis, D., Shaver, P. R. and Vernon, M. L. 'Physical, emotional and behavioral reactions to breaking up: The roles of gender, age, emotional involvement, and attachment style', *Personality and Social Psychology Bulletin*, 29(7) (2003), 871–84. doi:10.1177/0146167203029007006

[11]Wittstein, I., Thiemann, D. R. and Lima, J. A. C. 'Neurohumoral features of myocardial stunning due to sudden emotional stress', *ACC Current Journal Review*, 14(6) (2005), 6. doi:10.1016/j.accreview.2005.05.028

distressing death of a loved one. It is incredible, though, to know that medically this kind of impact can be triggered by loss. That, as sensational as it may sound, people really can collapse from a broken heart. I only include this condition to reassure you – if, like me, you spend a lot of time questioning your sanity when heartbroken – that on a scale from tiredness to full collapse, we are genuinely and scientifically affected by this loss.

The good news is that our hearts are not in medical-emergency levels of danger when we go through a break-up. We are wounded and not broken. While we can honestly say that on a neurological level we are in a state of mourning, we do not have to see this as either permanent or unfixable. In fact, one of the useful outcomes from studies on the bereavement-like state of heartbreak is that, unlike bereavement caused by a death, the loss of a romantic relationship is typically categorised as uncomplex rather than complex grief. This is not to say it isn't sad or difficult, but it is a transient state of grief. While the state we are thrown into may be similar and may elicit comparable symptoms to bereavement, recovery from heartbreak and the length of time this recovery takes is vastly better.[12] We can, however, still use the methods and advice often prescribed in cases of grief for the position we find ourselves in, as the support these techniques offer may help us to recover from heartbreak too.

Helping Us Along the Way

Grief is a complex thing, and it is now pretty widely acknowledged that the so-called stages of grief – denial, anger, bargaining, depression and acceptance – can happen to any degree, in any order and sometimes all at once. We may feel angry one minute, sad the next and then overwhelmed by a feeling of longing and loss. What a fun cocktail. It is helpful to look at small techniques we can use to ease the overall state of bereavement: things that may help to lift our moods while we essentially allow time to pass and let our minds process the change. If we can find ways to ease this transitional period a little, then at least we are helping ourselves as we grieve for the person and the relationship we have lost, rather than just enduring our pain.

[12]Biondi, M. and Picardi, A. 'Clinical and biological aspects of bereavement and loss-induced depression: A reappraisal', *Psychotherapy and Psychosomatics*, 65(5) (1996), 229–45. doi:10.1159/000289082

Some of the most uplifting studies I've read when looking at heartbreak as a kind of bereavement are those that track the impact of nature and the environment on grief and loss. These studies have a kind of beauty to them, as if somewhere, hidden in the world around us, are little antidotes waiting to help us and ease the symptoms we are battling. Research suggests that taking ourselves out into nature can actually decrease negative thoughts, lower our stress levels and ease symptoms of grief. It is not just some poetic fancy to go off and wander through the woods for the afternoon – it really can be a kind of medicine. In fact, in Japan, walking in the forest (or Shinrin-Yoku, translated as 'taking the atmosphere of the forest' or 'forest bathing') has been researched, funded and even prescribed by the Japanese government to the country's citizens for many years. Studies in Japan stretching back to the 1980s have shown that walking in a forest can lower blood pressure and cortisol levels, improve concentration and even boost the immune system due to the release of the chemical phytoncide from trees and plants.[13] Even now this practice is incorporated into the Japanese government's health programme, and in the United Kingdom it was recently proposed as an addition to the well-being list that GPs could officially recommend to patients.

---

[13]Hansen, M. M. et al. 'Shinrin-Yoku (forest bathing) and nature therapy: A state-of-the-art review', *International Journal of Environmental Research and Public Health*, 14(8) (2017), 851. doi:10.3390/ijerph14080851

Now, I am very much a city girl, born in London and currently still clinging on to living here despite every practical and financial challenge that involves, but I know that whenever I feel stressed or sad, a little voice in my head says 'I need to get out of the city.' What I find increasingly fascinating about the studies I read relating to our emotions is that so often the findings make me think 'Oh yeah, I've felt that/done that/instinctively been pulled towards that.' Very rarely do I read something and think it is a crazy theory that could only have come from a mad scientist up in their tower. I've wanted to take myself out into nature a hundred times when feeling low, but seeing the data that backs up this instinct makes me actually try to do it and find the time to schedule in that walk or trip. It stops me thinking of this desire as a whim or some kind of indulgence, and encourages me to listen to my need for natural surroundings and act on it.

In the next chapter there is more detail about the positive impact of exercise on the brain and how it can help to lift our mood and decrease our stress levels, but interestingly, in relation to nature, studies that have tracked groups walking in an urban environment or on a treadmill versus those walking in open green spaces record different degrees of this uplift.[14]

[14]Gladwell, V. F. et al. 'The great outdoors: How a green exercise environment can benefit all', *Extreme Physiology & Medicine*, 2(1) (2013), 3. doi:10.1186/2046-7648-2-3

It is not just that exercise helps to increase endorphins and decrease our cortisol and adrenaline levels, but that when this activity takes place in a natural environment the data shows a greater decrease in negative thought. A study at Carleton University in Ottawa tracked groups of students who were allocated different walking routes, one a green walk across campus and the other a walk through underpasses and tunnels designed to protect students from bad weather. The results showed that the green-space walking group were more positive and relaxed, and reported fewer negative emotions than the tunnel walkers. Their mood and mental state were affected not just by the exercise but by the environment.[15] So much of grief is about trying to alleviate negative thinking and lift the heavy sadness that comes along with it. If we can make even a small impact on this by going for a walk in some greenery, then that seems worth a try. Hopefully even those of us working in the darkest of office buildings or hunched over our kitchen tables can find a square or park somewhere to go for a walk in during our lunch breaks.

It is even possible, so scientists say, just to look at a little nature and feel some kind of lift. Maybe in addition to some time outdoors it is also time to surround ourselves with a few more plants and position our workstation closer to a window.

[15]Nisbet, E. K. and Zelenski, J. M. 'Underestimating nearby nature: Affective forecasting errors obscure the happy path to sustainability', *Psychological Science*, 22(9) (2011), 1101–6. doi:10.1177/0956797611418527

One regularly cited study from a Pennsylvania hospital showed that patients recovering from surgery had shorter post-operative hospital stays, received fewer negative evaluative comments in nurses' notes and took fewer potent analgesics when they had a room with a view of a natural environment than those patients whose windows looked onto a brick wall.[16] Patients healed a little better when they could see some trees, the study suggests. There are a great deal of studies in this area, but to take some tips from a recent study at the University of Michigan, even just twenty minutes in nature may help lift our moods. In this study the time spent in a natural environment was in no way aerobic and only immersive, and the results showed that over an eight-week period, a routine of three weekly sessions in nature had a positive hormonal impact on the participants.[17]

In addition to the studies that look at the soothing effects of nature, there are those that track the change of focus that comes from these natural surroundings. The activity of going for a walk in the woods, for example, is not just about being among the trees but about being somewhere that needs less scrutiny and thought than our daily lives.

[16]Ulrich, R. S. 'View through a window may influence recovery from surgery', *Science*, 224(4647) (1984), 420–1. doi:10.1126/science.6143402

[17]Hunter, M. R., Gillespie, B. W. and Chen, S. Y. 'Urban nature experiences reduce stress in the context of daily life based on salivary biomarkers', *Frontiers in Psychology*, 10 (2019), 722. doi:10.3389/fpsyg.2019.00722

There is not the same need for concentration in a natural environment and we do not have to engage our complete attention in the same way as when working in an office, for instance. Studies suggest that this allows for attention restoration and recovery from mental fatigue.[18] What we are engaging in, perhaps without actively meaning to, is a kind of mindfulness exercise, which can be another helpful technique to use when we are trying to process loss.

Many bereavement charities now promote meditation, mindfulness and breathing exercises as ways of processing grief, and while the benefits are of course subjective, there are more and more scientific studies that show a real correlation between the use of meditation and mindfulness and changes in our brains. A substantial review of meditation programmes used for psychological stress and well-being, undertaken in 2014 and looking at studies that included over 3,000 participants, found that data taken from these various studies showed positive effects from meditation techniques for both anxiety and depression.[19] This is not to say that these exercises are going to cure everything instantly, but these studies suggest that they can have a real impact on the kind of mild depression that accompanies heartbreak. I do

[18]Herzog, T. R., Maguire, C. P. and Nebel, M. B. 'Assessing the restorative components of environments', *Journal of Environmental Psychology*, 23(2) (2003), 159–70. doi: 10.1016/S0272-4944(02)00113-5

[19]Goyal, M. et al. 'Meditation programs for psychological stress and well-being: A systematic review and meta-analysis', *JAMA Internal Medicine*, 174(3) (2014), 357–68. doi:10.1001/jamainternmed.2013.13018

not use 'mild' to belittle how low you may be feeling but just to distinguish, as these studies do, depression linked to a sad event from the more serious condition of clinical, long-term depression. Now, a small note here, as full-on depression is such a hard condition to endure and clinical depression can sometimes be induced from grief: in the first few difficult weeks it may be a good idea to monitor just how low or depressed you feel. Typically, doctors use experiencing over two weeks of extreme low mood as a marker for more serious depression, so if that is where you think you are, you should always go and see a professional.

If you are looking for techniques to use at home rather than something a doctor may suggest, here is a simple one from a bereavement charity. This is a mindful breathing exercise, which ultimately has the aim of allowing you to feel calmer and to relax your mind. All you have to do is focus on the rise and fall of your chest as you breathe, paying attention to the air in your nostrils and the warmth of the breath as it leaves your body.[20] It sounds so minimal to do something like this in the grand scheme of all we are feeling, but this really is how simple mindfulness is. It is about concentrating on something like our breath and allowing our mind to relax

[20]Pritchard, S. '3 Ways to Use Mindfulness During Your Grief', Hospice of the Red River Valley. Available at: <https://www.hrrv.org/blog/3-ways-to-use-mindfulness-during-your-grief/>

as it moves away from complex, busy thoughts. The aim of these exercises in relation to grief is not to actually diminish the pain associated with a loss, but to acknowledge and process it.

If, like me, the simplicity of mindfulness makes you feel a tad sceptical, let me back it up with a little science. A recent study that investigated correlations between mindfulness and rejection showed that participants in the study who were asked to perform a mindfulness exercise before testing showed lower activation in the left ventrolateral prefrontal cortex during a rejection episode than those who did not use the technique.[21] This brain region is apparently associated with the inhibition of negative affect, meaning the suppression of negative emotions and poor self-perception. The subjects who practised mindfulness in this experiment experienced less activation in this region (i.e. they experienced fewer negative emotions that needed to be suppressed) during rejection than those who had not. MRI scans also showed less connectivity between this area of the brain and the bilateral amygdala and dorsal anterior cingulate cortex, suggesting that less social distress was created and less emotional pain was experienced by the subject. The brain

[21]Martelli, A. M., Chester, D. S., Brown, K. W., Eisenberger, N. I. and DeWall, C. N. 'When less is more: Mindfulness predicts adaptive affective responding to rejection via reduced prefrontal recruitment', *Social Cognitive and Affective Neuroscience*, 13(6) (2018), 648–55. doi:10.1093/scan/nsy037

did not have to battle the same intensity of negative affect when mindfulness had been used. So even if all these cortices and amygdalas may sound a little much, what even us laypeople can understand is that the brain behaved in a different way when mindfulness was used than when it was not, to the degree that it showed up on an MRI. Rejection and the pain it causes are such a huge part of the loss and grief we experience when we are heartbroken. If using mindfulness and meditation can alleviate this, it must be worth a try. Research has also found correlations between the use of these practices and a decrease in self-judgement[22] and an increase in self-kindness[23] – both things that sound very helpful to me right now. If doing these exercises can not only help us to process our loss but also ease the pain of rejection and encourage a little more self-kindness, imagine what a combination we could potentially achieve by using these techniques to help us heal.

Acquiring some tools to help us through grief – heartbreak-related or otherwise – can only be a positive gain. We will never get through life without loss, so it's useful to find some

---

[22]Doll, A., Holzel, B., Boucard, C. C., Wohlschläger, A. M. and Sorg, C. 'Mindfulness is associated with intrinsic functional connectivity between default mode and salience networks', *Frontiers in Human Neuroscience*, 9 (2015), 461. doi:10.3389/fnhum.2015.00461

[23]Parrish, M., Boyle, C. C., Dutcher, J. M, Bower, J. and Eisenberger, N. 'T87. Mindfulness training increases intrinsic connectivity between the default mode and frontoparietal control networks: Positive consequences for self-kindness in breast cancer survivors', *Biological Psychiatry*, 85(10) (2019), S162. doi:10.1016/j.biopsych.2019.03.410

techniques that work for each of us individually. The older we get, the more funerals we will go to – the more services, the more buffets, the more horrible logistical conversations about who is driving to or from the wake there will be – but although of course funerals are sad, they are also important and necessary and helpful. We know this: no matter how distressing we may find them, we know that culturally, socially and psychologically there is a reason we have them. We have, over time, built some kind of system for processing death. We have markers, events, anniversaries... We are allowed to recognise the loss and even have ceremonies associated with it.

We haven't really got there with heartbreak in the same way. There is no broken-heart ceremony. I may have had the odd heartbreak bonfire on the patio with my sister over the years, but this was always in secret and never because it was part of an official schedule. I think the grief of heartbreak can be murkier than other types of bereavement, even if it is not as severe, because of the lack of clear steps or protocol around it, which can make it much more confusing. For this reason, being kind to yourself and using coping mechanisms such as spending time outside in nature and taking time to let your mind rest are important practices to experiment with right now. And if, like me, you want to have a little patio bonfire, then I say go for it.

CHAPTER THREE

Ouch

There is something so gratifying about going to the doctor with an ailment you only suspect that you have and then hearing them pronounce a real and measurable diagnosis. Perhaps this says more about my sorry-to-bother-you approach to life than anything else, but there is always a niggling worry in my mind that either I am the cause of the problem or I am blowing it way out of proportion. I would love it if somehow a broken heart could be as provable and visual as a broken leg. I would like to hobble around on my broken heart and have people sign my cast with their good wishes. I could have X-rays and check-ups and be told that my fracture would take around six to eight weeks to heal.

The pain of heartache, though, is more obscure. It is not as visible or acknowledged; there is no broken-heart cast I have found as yet. This invisibility can make it more confusing and isolating when we feel this dreadful. I don't mean just feeling sad – we are probably pretty clear on that emotion right now, but it can be difficult to understand why in addition to everything else we feel like we've been kicked in the head. This is where modern science can be so brilliant and reassuring. We would not expect ourselves to bounce back from a broken leg. We would never try to go running the next day, or in my case probably ever. So it makes sense that step one in healing our broken hearts should be figuring out what kind of injury we have sustained.

How Heartbreak Hurts

There is a reason why all the poetic ways in which we talk about loss involve so many of the same adjectives we use to describe physical pain. We really are in pain. We really do ache. The symptoms of heartbreak go way beyond the clichéd weepy mess we may picture (sometimes accurately, in my case). A broken heart can affect our sleep, our immune function, our muscles and our digestion, to name but a few of the fun documented side effects. If we feel beaten up, it is not all in our head. We genuinely are a little beaten up right now. Not only have we incurred real injuries to our body from this unexpected kick in the gut, but the way our mind processes the emotional rejection we feel during heartbreak actually shares the same neural pathways as a physical injury.[24] The sadness, the aching, the heavy heart we are dragging around is activating the same part of the brain as physical, leg-in-a-cast-style pain.

The way we process a broken heart is not so different to the way we experience a physical injury. It is not the case that one is 'real' pain and one is not. Studies in this area have shown that when scanning the brains of heartbroken subjects and triggering their emotional pain, this stimulus lights up the same part of the brain that is activated by a physical injury[25] (the secondary somatosensory cortex and dorsal posterior insula, for those of you who want to know the exact place you are being punched right now). This is not true of every emotional reaction you could have in life but is specifically linked to rejection, the very thing we feel when we are heartbroken. A person or, in theory, a group of people choosing to leave you is represented in the

[24]Tchalova, K. and Eisenberger, N. I. 'How the brain feels the hurt of heartbreak: Examining the neurobiological overlap between social and physical pain', *Brain Mapping: An Encyclopedic Reference*, 3 (2015), 15–20. doi:10.1016/B978-0-12-397025-1.00144-5

[25]Kross, E., Berman M. G., Mischel, W., Smith, E. E. and Wager, T. D. 'Social rejection shares somatosensory representations with physical pain', *Proceedings of the National Academy of Sciences*, 108(15) (2011), 6270–5. doi:10.1073/pnas.1102693108

brain in the same way as physical pain. When heartbroken participants in these studies were, for example, shown photos of their ex-partners, the results on an MRI showed that the brain registered this pain in the same way it would a physical trauma. Professor Naomi Eisenberger at UCLA is my new hero in this area. She investigates social exclusion and romantic rejection, scanning brains as often as I'm sure Sarah does, and revealing how our minds experience this type of emotional injury.[26] Not only does Eisenberger's research show that physical pain and social pain rely on shared neural substrates, meaning that they use the same parts of our central nervous system, but she also explores why this happens: why we would have this kind of painful alarm system in our minds when experiencing rejection.[27] Physical pain is activated in our brains to protect us, giving us a sharp warning that something is causing us harm. Eisenberger's research suggests that humans developed this neural overlap of social rejection and physical pain because both represent an evolutionary threat.[28] Social exclusion or rejection could be as dangerous for us on an evolutionary level as, say, hyperthermia or starvation, or in theory could actually lead to these very states. Our brains use the same

---

[26]Eisenberger, N. I. 'The neural bases of social pain: Evidence for shared representations with physical pain', *Psychosomatic Medicine*, 74(2) (2012),126–35. doi: 10.1097/PSY.0b013e3182464dd1

[27]Eisenberger, N. I., Lieberman, M. D. and Williams, K. D. 'Does rejection hurt? An fMRI study of social exclusion', *Science*, 302(5643) (2003), 290–2. doi:10.1126/science.1089134

[28]Eisenberger, N. I. and Lieberman, M. D. 'Why rejection hurts: A common neural alarm system for physical and social pain', *Trends in Cognitive Sciences*, 8(7) (2004), 294–300. doi:10.1016/j.tics.2004.05.010

neurochemical and neural substrates to create an alert for us, to cause us 'pain', in order to prevent the potentially harmful consequences of social separation. Our heartache is triggering the same reaction in our brains as a real, physical injury, meaning that rejection really does hurt.

The Break-Up Boxing Match

At the same time as enduring the pain of rejection, we are also likely to be recovering from a few other unpleasant side effects. Just as my stomach reacted badly when I had my worst ever heartbreak all those years ago, there are many other ways in which our bodies are affected when we are trying to recover from a broken heart. Many of these can be explained in the simplest terms by the impact of stress. The stress caused by the shock of our loss and rejection creates a real, physical blow to our bodies. The hit of cortisol, the main stress hormone in the body, which we receive when we experience a break-up, combined with the drop in dopamine and oxytocin (hormones typically in the brain when we experience feelings of love) can create a strong chemical cocktail.[29] This quick hormonal shift is one of the reasons we can feel so physically awful. Our muscles are one of the

[29]Bosch, O. J. and Young, L. J. 'Oxytocin and social relationships: From attachment to bond disruption'. In: Hurlemann, R. and Grinevich, V. (eds), *Behavioral Pharmacology of Neuropeptides: Oxytocin*. Cham: Springer (2017), 97–117. doi:10.1007/7854_2017_10

many areas affected. The brain sends cortisol to the muscles in preparation for 'fight-or-flight' mode, the reactive, protective state we are wired to enter when threatened in some way. Our brain, perceiving that we are in danger and may, literally, need to run, sends cortisol to the muscles to trigger them into a kind of 'ready-for-action' state. If we don't then instantly use our charged-up muscles to run or fight, this can leave them tensed up and taut, causing a range of side effects, including headaches, tightness in the chest, stiff necks and aching backs.[30]

Our broken hearts can also affect our stomachs, as I was lucky enough to find out. The focus the brain suddenly places on our muscles not only sends extra cortisol in their direction but also diverts blood away from the digestive system in order to make sure the muscles have adequate blood supply and are as strong as possible. This diversion can upset the stomach and digestive system, triggering cramps, diarrhoea or, in my case, the unprecedented sensation of appetite loss. The HPA axis, which Sarah referred to in our first conversation about my appetite, stands for the hypothalamic-pituitary-adrenal axis, and is perhaps not something we laypeople know that much about. It is essentially our central stress response system. When our brain becomes stressed by something physical

---

[30]Crofford, L. J. 'Chronic pain: Where the body meets the brain', *Transactions of the American Clinical and Climatological Association*, 126 (2015), 167–83.

or psychological, a domino effect occurs until the adrenal cortex (the final A in HPA) releases stress hormones in response. This mini series of smoke signals that go off inside us are all there for protection, to help us fight back against a perceived threat, but they are also disruptive – particularly if we are not going to actively defend ourselves in a physical way. Studies have even shown that stress can change the composition of our gut microbiota, also causing our digestion to work differently.[31]

Our immune system is another area that can take a beating. In the immediate aftermath of a break-up, the hit of cortisol we receive is not actually a negative hormone for our immunity. It is designed to push us into a kind of survival state and therefore, although causing some unpleasant side effects, is meant to help. There are different levels and types of stress, though, and studies in this area distinguish between so-called brief naturalistic stressors, which are in the moment or immediate – so something like sitting an exam – and so-called stressful event sequences, which are considered longer and prolonged stressful situations. One regularly cited example of the latter is being heartbroken, and it is this longer stressful state that can impair our health.[32] In the case of a broken

[31]Molina-Torres, G., Rodriguez-Arrastia, M., Roman, P., Sanchez-Labraca, N. and Cardona, D. 'Stress and the gut microbiota-brain axis', *Behavioural Pharmacology*, 30(2 and 3) (2019), 187–200. doi:10.1097/FBP.0000000000000478
[32]Segerstrom, S. C. and Miller, G. E. 'Psychological stress and the human immune system: A meta-analytic study of 30 years of inquiry', *Psychological Bulletin*, 130(4) (2004), 601–30. doi:10.1037/0033-2909.130.4.601

heart, we do not just receive a momentary hit of cortisol; it can be released and released and released as we continue to feel the stress of our loss for far longer than the actual event of the break-up. We are not just getting a rush of cortisol as we experience the initial shock, we are agonising and worrying and replaying the sadness of this event over and over in our minds, and so the release of cortisol keeps on coming. It isn't just performing its original task of getting us the hell out of there and away from that grizzly bear, but instead it is being released for longer than its initial purpose, and this can start to upset and even overwhelm our health.[33]

It feels instinctive to most of us that as we get tired and stressed, we can end up getting sick. The state we are in when recovering from a break-up can be a heightened version of this. Depending on how your body reacts to stress, and the levels of cortisol hitting you right now, your immune system could be taking quite the broken-heart beating. Studies looking at stress caused by the loss of a partner have shown repeatedly that participants experience a decline in natural killer cell cytotoxicity[34] – meaning that when we are heartbroken we do not have the same stuff to fight off infection that we usually have. I do not mean to say all this

[33]Sapolsky, R. M. *Why Zebras Don't Get Ulcers: An Updated Guide to Stress, Stress-Related Disease, and Coping.* New York: Freeman, 1998.

[34]Irwin, M., Daniels, M., Risch, S. C., Bloom, E. and Weiner, H. 'Plasma cortisol and natural killer cell activity during bereavement', *Biological Psychiatry*, 24(2) (1988), 173–8. doi:10.1016/0006-3223(88)90272-7

to make you feel worse but to reassure you that there is a real, documented reason for feeling this dreadful. On so many levels, a broken heart really can affect our health. It can cause our immune function to struggle, it can make our bodies ache, it can cause headaches and colds or even the occasional glamorous dose of break-up diarrhoea. We do not have to ask apologetically for a real diagnosis here. We have a diagnosis: we are heartbroken, and that is real enough.

Helping Us Along the Way

One of the areas of neuroscience that Sarah researches is interoception, meaning our ability to read the internal workings of our bodies. So often when I've talked to her about heartbreak, she has referred to studies in this area. Interoception is not just about our bodies giving us basic physical cues, such as telling us when we are hungry or thirsty; it also affects the link we have to our emotions and our minds. Research shows that those of us who are more able to read the internal workings of our bodies, for instance accurately detecting the beat of our hearts or the waves of our stomachs, also experience our emotions more intensely.[35]

[35]Critchley, H. D. and Garfinkel, S. N. 'Interoception and emotion', *Current Opinion in Psychology*, 17 (2017), 7–14. doi:10.1016/j.copsyc.2017.04.020

Participants in one of Sarah's studies who were undergoing therapy for fear of spiders were shown to be more successful in overcoming that fear if they were also more successful at listening to the internal physical workings of their bodies.[36] Those reading their bodies clearly – in this experiment, those with higher accuracy results on detecting their heartbeats – could also read their emotions more clearly. These types of studies suggest that if we are able to listen to our bodies successfully we may also be able to listen more accurately to our minds. Research in this area even suggests that our decision-making (or 'gut instinct') is stronger when we are more able to listen to our bodies. Our ability to make intuitive decisions is hindered when we can't read our bodies and helped when we can.[37] Although merely acknowledging our aches and pains may not feel like the quick fix we crave at the moment, it really can help just to listen and react to our body's signals. If we try to understand a little more about the impact our heartbreak has had on us, we can get a little closer to recovery. It can help to scan through our body and think about the signals it is giving us. It may be that your achy back, which has suddenly twinged out of nowhere, is not actually such a mystery.

[36]Watson, D. R, Garfinkel, S. N, Gould van Praag, C. et al. 'Computerized exposure therapy for spider phobia: Effects of cardiac timing and interoceptive ability on subjective and behavioral outcomes', *Psychosomatic Medicine*, 81(1) (2019), 90–9. doi:10.1097/PSY.0000000000000646

[37]Dunn, B. D, Galton, H. C., Morgan, R., Evans, D., Oliver, C., Meyer, M., Cusack, R., Lawrence, A. D. and Dalgleish, T. 'Listening to your heart: How interoception shapes emotion experience and intuitive decision making', *Psychological Science*, 21(12) (2010), 1835–44. doi:10.1177/0956797610389191

In addition to seeking help for stiff necks or back spasms, we can also do things to release stress and decrease the cortisol that may be affecting us. When I'm at my lowest, tears burst out of me at the most inconvenient times. I have cried on buses, in bathrooms, at home, at the office – probably in other people's homes and at other people's offices. I used to have a trick where I thought really hard about an Ali G sketch where he got angry about the deception of the Wonderbra in order to stop tears piling up at awkward moments. When you are heartbroken it can be exhausting feeling so sad. You are either crying, trying not to cry or drained from all the crying yesterday. I know crying all the time might not seem super fun at the moment, but there is a reason we are doing that a lot right now. Crying actually helps release stress and expel cortisol; it is one of the many clever ways in which our bodies help us to recover from distress. Studies have even shown that there are different kinds of tears and, incredibly, emotional tears contain higher levels of stress hormones, releasing more cortisol from our bodies. It is not merely crying that releases stress – you can't just poke yourself in the eye and hope that as they water you will start to feel better – you must be crying from emotion specifically. Emotional tears contain more mood-regulating manganese, helping to activate the parasympathetic nervous system and restore the body to a state of balance.[38] How clever the body is. We are genuinely crying out the stress we feel, expelling the excess hormones that have disrupted our systems, shedding them out through our tears. So allowing ourselves to cry can not only help to mend our broken hearts but can ease the pressure on our bodies too.

There is also the incredible power of exercise. The proven benefits of exercise for stress levels are pretty universally acknowledged, so although it may feel hard to get up and out when we are exhausted and sad, the advantages really are worth it. I know, I know, this feels like you're a teenager being told by your parents to get out of bed on a Sunday morning. Everything about being heartbroken makes us want to curl up and hibernate, but exercise really can make us feel better. If you will not listen to me, then listen to the neuroscientists. Studies show that if we exercise even a few times a week, our endorphin levels increase and our cortisol and adrenaline levels go down. A major review of this area of research showed that when looking at data from nearly 20,000 participants there was roughly a 40% reduction in stress and anxiety following physical activity.[39] There have

[38]Bylsma, L. M., Gračanin, A. and Vingerhoets, A. J. J. M. 'The neurobiology of human crying', *Clinical Autonomic Research*, 29(1) (2019), 63–73. doi:10.1007/s10286-018-0526-y

[39]Hamer, M., Stamatakis, E. and Steptoe, A. 'Dose-response relationship between physical activity and mental health', *British Journal of Sports Medicine*, 43(14) (2008), 1111–4. doi:10.1136/bjsm.2008.046243

been more recent studies showing that aerobic exercise even reduces symptoms of post-traumatic stress.[40] Trying to do some form of exercise that elevates our heart rate and decreases our cortisol levels is an active way we can help our broken hearts and ease the symptoms we are currently dealing with.

It is a little unfair that our broken hearts are not exactly visible injuries, but if this *were* a broken leg, or a cold, or some other clearly defined illness, I know that we would all be taking our medicine and our vitamins and listening to our physiotherapists. This may not be us at our sexiest or strongest and, yes, this list of ways that heartbreak messes with our bodies is not hugely attractive, but how much better it is to know that this is happening. How much better to understand the many ways you could be affected right now. Maybe you only have mild versions of these symptoms, maybe you didn't even realise that any of these sensations could be connected to your break-up in the first place, but the world of science tells us that these reactions really do occur. They exist to the point that they can be counted and measured and scanned and researched. You could even go wild and make a pie chart or two if you were so inclined.

[40]Fetzner, M. G. and Asmundson, G. J. G. 'Aerobic exercise reduces symptoms of posttraumatic stress disorder: A randomized controlled trial', *Cognitive Behaviour Therapy*, 44(4) (2015), 301–13. doi:10.1080/16506073.2014.916745

The benefit of seeing these symptoms as real, as the result of measurable hormone levels and reactions in our bodies that have been caused by heartbreak, is that we can also have faith that these levels will readjust. We can even take action ourselves to help those shifts take place and to help us feel better. We can aid our recovery and mend our broken hearts by looking at these slightly unpleasant symptoms and counteracting them. I realise this is not a hugely fun task and I don't spout all this advice as someone who thinks it is easy, but it is *possible*, so it is worth a try. I am with you, I am on your side and I am signing your broken-heart cast with all my best wishes.

CHAPTER FOUR

When You Can't Find Your Marbles

I still have a password on my Facebook account that I asked my sister to set for me over fifteen years ago, at the time making her promise not to tell me what it was, because when utterly heartbroken and feeling insane I would keep logging in to see what my heartbreaker was doing. I don't know what I hoped to find on there, but I fell into a kind of irrational cyber-world loop. I do not need that level of intervention anymore, thank goodness, and am able to set my own internet passwords, but because I never changed my login details on that account, whenever I have to type those same letters into the password field it reminds me of how lost I felt back then. I don't think I am an obsessive person – I'd never shown signs of that kind of behaviour before. I like to think my love of science makes me fundamentally quite a rational being. But this was like I had morphed into someone I'd seen in trashy movies. I was suddenly this clichéd dumped woman – it was a bizarre thing to experience. Where had my brain gone? Where was my normal personality? Was I going insane?

Are We Crazy?

I should start here by saying that no neuroscientist would use the term crazy, nor would any psychologist or counsellor or professional of any kind, and I am certainly not labelling you as such myself. I am just posing the question that I know was going round my mind at that time and may well be going round yours. In the last chapter we looked at the more physical effects of heartbreak on the body, but what about its impact on our mental state? Or in my case, what had turned my usually rational brain into such an obsessive, needy mess? Had my mind been altered in some way?

Well, it turns out that according to research in this area, yes, it had – and not just by the break-up but by being in love at all. Studies show that when we are in love our brains are significantly affected, even suggesting there are love-related alterations in the very architecture of our brains.

These changes do not completely vanish even when we are no longer in that relationship.[41] When we are in love we are hit by the chemical oxytocin (otherwise known as the love hormone), which triggers a series of hormonal reactions and physical side effects, and stimulates a particular kind of brain activity.[42] One of the main parts of the brain activated by this is the reward centre, causing a drive to be ignited inside us that alters our previously neutral state and pushes us to form a connection with the person we now adore.

Just as love significantly affects our brains, so too does heartbreak. Studies have shown that when we are heartbroken the impact on that same reward centre has a very different and significant outcome. Brain scans of heartbroken participants actually mirror those of people in withdrawal from marijuana, cocaine and even heroin. We are pushed into a state of chemical withdrawal and, incredibly, experience the same regional brain activity as someone fighting drug addiction. That is how intense a hit our minds have taken. It is not that we have had some single-white-female personality shift, it is that our brains are now experiencing the same kinds of cravings as a drug addict scanning for a fix.

---

[41]Song, H., Zou, Z., Kou, J. et al. 'Love-related changes in the brain: A resting-state functional magnetic resonance imaging study', *Frontiers in Human Neuroscience, 9* (2015), 71. doi:10.3389/fnhum.2015.00071
[42]MacGill, M. 'What is the link between love and oxytocin?', Medical News Today (4 September 2017). Available at: <https://www.medicalnewstoday.com/articles/275795>

Cravings and Comedowns

With the benefit of hindsight and of scientific data, that manic energy I felt when heartbroken no longer seems quite as bizarre as I first thought. If my brain when heartbroken looks even marginally like that of someone in heroin withdrawal, then logging into Facebook a few times suddenly does not seem quite as embarrassing or extreme. The more research that is done on the brain when in love and when in its post-love recovery, the more sense it makes that we end up on such a rollercoaster.

Firstly, you have the experience of falling in love in the first place. Scientists studying the effects of love on the brain have recorded two main regions that appear affected when we are in love: the ventral tegmental area, or VTA to its friends, and the caudate.[43] The caudate is thought to be responsible for the 'rush' sensation you experience when in love, aiding love's addictive quality. This region is located in a central position within the brain, forming connections to many other areas such as the reward centre, the memory and the cerebral cortex where we do our thinking. Studies tracking the activation of the caudate in relation to love

---

[43]Xu, X., Aron, A., Brown, L., Cao, G., Feng, T. and Weng, X. 'Reward and motivation systems: A brain mapping study of early-stage intense romantic love in Chinese participants', *Human Brain Mapping*, 32(2) (2011), 249–57. doi:10.1002/hbm.21017

(for example, when showing participants images of their romantic partners) suggest that this centrally connected region of the brain pulls together many strands during the in-love state, and this is why you get an intense hit of romantic passion or a kind of ecstatic rush. The other region, the VTA, is part of the brain's reward system – the area that generates pleasure and motivation. It manufactures dopamine, the chemical that gives you not only a sensation of ecstasy but also energy, drive and focus, propelling you to keep pursuing that mate and gaining those hits of reward and pleasure. It is also the area of the brain that is activated by cocaine. One theory is that love is not exactly an emotion in the same way as fear, sadness or joy, but is in fact a mammalian drive that is designed to make us pursue a mate.[44] This could be why it is so intertwined with the reward centre of the brain.

When we are heartbroken, the regions of the brain previously being stimulated during our loved-up state do not do what we might expect. They do not instantly calm down or decrease arousal; instead, they remain activated. Not to sound like a petulant child, but this just seems really unfair. Why not switch these activated regions off and give us a break when we are heartbroken? Why do

44Fisher, H. E. 'Lust, attraction, and attachment in mammalian reproduction', *Human Nature*, 9 (1998), 23–52. doi:10.1007/s12110-998-1010-5

we remain in a state of love when we no longer have a lover? Studies have shown that part of the initial struggle of being heartbroken is that the regions within the brain activated by love are still working away. We are still propelled to pursue that mate. We are still receiving the same brain signals. Brain scans of rejected lovers showed that the VTA was still lit up after the break-up, as was the ventral pallidum, a brain region linked to feelings of deep attachment.[45] We are, ultimately, still in love, even if we have the logical information that we are no longer in a relationship.

As we start to process our heartbreak, our brains begin to battle withdrawal and all the challenges of addiction. This revolves around the nucleus accumbens – the brain region linked with not only the sensations of wanting and craving but also focus and determination. We are not even burnt-out addicts right now. We are motivated. We are energised. We are ready to stay up all night scrolling through social media. We are driven to keep finding ways to activate that reward centre, even when the person previously triggering it is no longer there.

[45]Fisher, H. E., Brown, L. L., Aron, A., Strong, G. and Mashek, D. 'Reward, addiction, and emotion regulation systems associated with rejection in love', *Journal of Neurophysiology*, 104(1) (2010), 51–60. doi:10.1152/jn.00784.2009

I know this isn't exactly painting a pretty picture, but the important takeaway is that you are not feeling this way because you are weak or crazy or losing your mind. If you feel driven towards some out-of-character behaviour right now, there is a clear scientific reason for it. Your brain is genuinely struggling with a form of chemical withdrawal, so please be kind to your mind and to yourself. No name-calling. No saying you are crazy. Your brain may be in a battle at the moment, but it is not going insane. No one would expect a heroin addict to bounce back right away, so let's take these insights as an important starting point for our recovery. Yes, we want to kick the habit, but let's take a moment to acknowledge what our brains are going through. Our context here is one of addiction and withdrawal.

I wish all those years ago I had known that my brain was being affected in this way, both in my loved-up state and afterwards. If I hadn't had a neuroscientist for a best friend and hadn't bugged her constantly for articles and studies and facts about heartbreak, I think I would still be doubting my own sanity even now. It does make sense on an evolutionary level that love, partnership and ultimately, I suppose, procreation would be encouraged and rewarded within our physiological make-up. I would not have guessed, though, that the after-effects of losing those rewards would be so fundamentally difficult to recover from.

Thankfully, scientists studying broken-hearted subjects like you and me do not spend all their time identifying problems – sometimes they work on testing out some helpful solutions too. So let's start our attempt at rehab with a little scientific advice.

Helping Us Along the Way

Happily, recent research into a variety of cognitive strategies for helping people recover from a broken heart and its addictive after-effects has shown positive results. One successful strategy, also used to help reduce cravings in other forms of addiction, is the technique of distraction: forcing your mind to another topic or activity any time it wanders towards the thing you are craving. Now, bear with me for a moment as I know this may not sound like the magic-pill solution you were hoping for, but what is so reassuring about this study is that the use of distraction to recover from heartbreak showed significant results and decreased emotional pain. This is not just some well-meaning friend sitting across the table and suggesting you 'try not to think about your ex' while you, naturally, want to throw a heavy object at their head. These are positive findings from an impartial group of scientists who have found success when using this strategy.

Researchers from the Neurocognition of Emotion and Motivation Lab at the University of Missouri–St. Louis measured the intensity of emotional responses from their participants when shown photos of their ex-partners, using electrodes placed on the posterior of the scalp. These electrodes took something called an EEG reading: a measurement that records not only emotion but motivated attention, meaning how captivated the person was by the photo they were shown. The researchers also measured how positive and negative the participants felt about their ex-partners and how much love they still felt using a scale and a questionnaire. The EEG data taken from the participants when using distraction techniques – in this experiment they had to think through a series of questions and answers about favourite foods, movies, holidays and so on in order to redirect their minds elsewhere – showed that the subjects felt better than before they adopted this approach.[46] Their well-being was higher and their recovery more progressed. It did not decrease their feelings of love for their ex-partner, but it did help with the negative emotions caused by the loss of love. It is not that distraction stops you feeling in love, but this study suggests that it can help you stop feeling quite so dreadful about the heartbreak. This technique is more about easing the level of distress so that, as time passes and that distress starts to drop, you have not endured as tough a period and are more positive, more capable and more able to move on. Distraction techniques are even used in cases of PTSD, anxiety and, in some studies, chronic pain.[47] Not only does research show that distraction helps decrease self-reported negative emotion but MRI scans of people using these techniques show real variations in brain activity and decreased activation in the amygdala.[48] Amygdala activity is thought to signal the degree to which a stimulus, so a thought or an image, requires some sort of further processing – whether it's to bring this stimulus into focal attention, to prepare a response to it or to enhance it further into our memory.

[46]Langeslag, S. J. E. and Sanchez, M. E. 'Down-regulation of love feelings after a romantic break-up: Self-report and electrophysiological data', *Journal of Experimental Psychology: General*, 147(5) (2018), 720–33. doi:10.1037/xge0000360

[47]Moyal, N., Henik, A. and Anholt, G. E. 'Cognitive strategies to regulate emotions – current evidence and future directions', *Frontiers in Psychology*, 4 (2014), 1019. doi:10.3389/fpsyg.2013.01019

[48]McRae, K., Hughes, B., Chopra, S., Gabrieli, J. D., Gross, J. J. and Ochsner, K. N. 'The neural bases of distraction and reappraisal', *Journal of Cognitive Neuroscience*, 22(2) (2010), 248–62. doi:10.1162/jocn.2009.21243

The decreased activity in this area of the brain when using distraction is a fascinating representation of how our focus has been changed and how the area of the brain used for attention has been genuinely affected.

If 'distraction' feels a little vague right now, then here are some practical suggestions from scientists at the University of Toledo.[49] You can use more active distraction techniques, such as exercise, watching a movie, listening to music, cleaning and tidying or going for a walk – these are all activities you can throw yourself into as thoughts you are trying to avoid recur. Or, if you find your mind is wandering a lot at work or at times you can't instantly go out to a spin class, here are some slightly quieter options. You can try counting backwards from twenty; you can focus on your breathing and move your mind away from your thoughts; you can do some kind of puzzle like a short Sudoku or crossword; even just doodling on a piece of paper has been shown to help. Another helpful technique that can be used anywhere and at any time (no pens, paper or Sudoku needed) is simply to focus your attention on the environment around you, for example looking around the room and noting all the colours you can see, or counting all the things that are blue, or listening until you can name five different sounds.

---

[49]Tull, M. 'Using Distraction for Coping With Emotions and PTSD', Verywell Mind (September 2019). Available at: <https://www.verywellmind.com/coping-with-emotions-with-distraction-2797606>

These ideas may sound trite, but they all actively take your mind away from its current thoughts, and that is what can genuinely help. Any short, focused exercise – similar to many mindfulness techniques – which helps you concentrate on something other than thoughts of your heartbreaker can help you recover. Studies around the use of mindfulness have shown that the restorative effects of these practices on the brain have had therapeutic effects on addictive behaviour.[50]

It may be that you have already tried to distract yourself without realising it. There is an understandable tendency to try to just shake off thoughts about your ex-partner – I think to some degree we probably all attempt this. What we might not realise is that it really is actively helpful and worth trying. An interesting finding in this area of research is that our ability to suppress unwanted thoughts is significantly impaired when we are tired.[51] We just don't have the same strength or ability when we have not had enough sleep, and those unwanted thoughts, or thoughts we are trying to distract ourselves from, creep in much more easily. If you are struggling with distraction techniques, consider your sleep patterns and tiredness levels as you will find them much harder if you are exhausted. This is another great motivator

[50]Garland, E. L., Bryan, M. A., Hanley, A. W. and Howard, M. O. 'Neurocognitive mechanisms of mindfulness-based interventions for addiction'. In: Verdejo-Garcia, A. (ed.), *Cognition and Addiction*. Cambridge, MA: Academic Press, 2020, 283–93.

[51]Van Schie, K. and Anderson, M. C. 'Successfully controlling intrusive memories is harder when control must be sustained', *Memory*, 25(9) (2017), 1201–16. doi:10.1080/09658211.2017.1282518

to try to get enough rest. Sleep disturbance, as we know, is a bereavement-like symptom that is often triggered by the grief of heartbreak, and it's well worth seeking help for this problem as you will be significantly stronger and more able to keep yourself actively distracted if you are well-rested.[52]

A second helpful finding from research carried out at the University of Missouri–St. Louis was in the area of negative reappraisal as a coping strategy when heartbroken. The men and women taking part in the study, who were all suffering from the pain of a recent break-up, were asked to think of the things they didn't like about their ex-partners, and to actively focus on any negatives they could find whenever their minds drifted towards thoughts about that person. This too might be something we have half-heartedly tried ourselves, or even had friends suggest we do when we are wailing 'But he had such strong arms!' at them while crying into our sangria. How often have friends tried to rally a little energy or fight inside us by listing all our ex's faults? But this research suggests that this can be more than a desperate attempt by our friends to cheer us up; this really is a technique we can use to help ourselves recover. If we try to redirect our minds towards the negative – even

---

[52]If you're struggling with sleep and looking for some help, you can find useful advice in Lucinda Ford's *How to Sleep*, published in the same series as this book. See Ford, L. *How to Sleep: A Natural Method*. Oxford: Fairlight Books, 2019.

negative things that seem silly or small – this can have an impact on the way we feel about the person we have lost, and can even help decrease the intensity of our feelings. This in turn can help us move on from being mentally stuck in the 'in love' state and make progress towards recovery. According to the EEG readings in this study, this technique helped decrease participants' emotional responses to their ex, as with distraction, but also helped decrease feelings of love. Focusing on someone's flaws may seem like a petty exercise (I'm sure when this break-up first occurred we didn't imagine that we would be sitting at home listing how our exes used too many emojis or flossed at the breakfast table), but at the moment our brains are unfairly trapped. Even if it seems silly, in order to help ease our minds out of this position, it is worth giving this technique a try. We are not destroying that person or their reputation in reality – you can keep this list as private as you like – we are just helping to counteract the bias fuelled by addiction. Our minds have been in shock, denial and pain, and yet still the chemical and hormonal impact of love can keep us from starting to feel better again. So make that list, mental or otherwise, and use it when you need to. Every little annoying thing, every little flaw.

One warning from this study is that focusing on negative thoughts *generally* can, understandably, affect our mood. So the time to use this technique is when our mind drifts towards how incredible the person we have lost is, rather than all the time. When we think about their handsome face, we need to redirect our minds towards their smelly feet. You don't want to be walking around constantly thinking about a list of their annoying traits, or you might end up feeling pretty miserable, but as a balancing technique it can achieve real results.

Until I read these studies, I was pretty sure the strongest addiction I had ever been affected by was my emotionally charged relationship with coffee. I was late to start drinking the stuff and so my theory is that I am making up for lost time. (Please note, this has not been scientifically proven.) The more I read about the addiction-like qualities of heartbreak, though, and the more I look back on what I now realise were recovery periods for me, the more I can see that coffee has not been my only drug. Love is powerful and an incredibly hard thing to wean ourselves off. If I ever try to break up with coffee, at least now I know that distraction and negative reappraisal will be my tools, and if I start pressing my face against coffee shop windows I will know why. As we attempt to recover from this difficult period, let's try to remember how powerful addiction is and not beat ourselves up on top of enduring the battle we are fighting. A little kindness eases everything.

CHAPTER FIVE

The Art of Solitude

Solitude and loneliness are not the same thing. Solitude is something we can all enjoy at times – loneliness, though, is a whole different monster. We might relish our alone time, but who wants to say they are lonely? What kind of rebranding genius would we need in order to make lonely sound cool or even acceptable? And yet when we are heartbroken, loneliness can appear from nowhere and can, unfairly, be one of the harder side effects of this whole rollercoaster to actually identify.

In my twenties I moved to New York to do an internship. This was as glamorous an opportunity as I could ever have imagined. I had grown up in London so New York, as spellbinding as it seemed, did not scare me in the big-city sense, and I was completely unprepared to feel anything other than happy and excited every second I was there. I was so used to telling everyone how fortunate I was that it didn't occur to me that I was struggling. 'It's amazing, I'm so lucky,' I would say. 'I think I spend a lot of time alone? And that I often feel quite alone? But that's fine. I don't mind! I am sleeping a lot, because I guess I'm really tired… but I have more time to sleep because I don't know that many people. I see what people are doing on social media, though. I'm fine. I'm really lucky!'

It was only through talking to my wise neuroscientist chum that I started to become aware of how different what I was feeling and what I was saying really were. Sarah would repeat back to me the things I was saying, and they didn't sound quite the same coming from her as they had inside my head. These were the days of dial-up phone cards with scratch-off login codes. I would stand on a street corner and call Sarah from a payphone, my view of New York as beautiful as in any movie, and yet our conversation would be about how I had two friends and went to bed at nine. My reality versus the way it must have looked from the outside were so different. It was only through saying how I felt out loud that I could see I wasn't just spending time alone – I was lonely. I wasn't checking social media for fun; I was feeling isolated and homesick.

It is very easy to miss the signs of loneliness, and the depression that can accompany it, when it sneaks up on you gradually or appears in a place where you least expect it. How could I feel lonely somewhere as vibrant and beautiful as New York? There were people everywhere. I was lucky that Sarah could ask me the questions she did and help me to clarify what I was feeling. It is hard to do this for ourselves, though, and we are not always lucky enough to have someone there at exactly the right time to point it out. My New York experience was a little like a break-up. I went from being in my home city with lots of friends and my family nearby to somewhere where I hardly knew anyone. That kind of sudden change can be unsettling, and when we are reeling from a break-up we can be a little paralysed at first from the shock of suddenly being by ourselves.

Am I Alone Now?

I know that most scientists, therapists and professionals are very careful to frame their ideas and research with an element of delicacy. Every study I read seems to *imply* something rather than *prove* it, and I understand that this is a very sensible way to speak when you are a genius scientist and held in great esteem. As a non-scientist, though, I would like to give the following response to the question above: Nope! No! You are not alone! Do not worry! Single and alone are not the same thing. Maybe you have gone from living with someone to living alone, or maybe there are things you are doing now by yourself that you used to do with another person, but there are many types of relationships, many forms of community and many ways of feeling connected to others. Loneliness and isolation are challenging symptoms that may come from a break-up, but we do not need to label ourselves in a new, negative way on top of struggling with these feelings. Single is different to alone; single can be great (even if it may not feel that way right now) – it is loneliness and isolation that we need to be careful of.

The shift from being in a couple to being single can be difficult, of course, and it is with this shift that we may need some help. We often hear people say that it feels like a part of them is missing when they have become single or lost someone. Well, research suggests that in a relationship we connect on more than just an emotional level, and that suddenly being without that other person can have a significant impact on us. Did you know that scientists studying the biological rhythms and cycles of couples can actually see measurable ways that their bodies synchronise when they are in a relationship? And that on top of this we can be affected by even short separations, let alone a sudden and permanent break-up? Studies into the physiological effect of partner separations have shown that even during four-to-seven-day separations there is a measurable change in couples' HPA axis activity and cortisol levels, which can have an impact on sleep, anxiety and stress levels.[53] Of course we are also affected by habit, routine and social plans all changing, but those losses we can see more plainly. At the same time, on a much less visible level, we are experiencing the impact of the day-to-day absence of that person.

Broken Connections

If being single all of a sudden has left you feeling destabilised and unsettled, science suggests that this could be about more than just the loss of love. Research shows that, incredibly, our body actually syncs up with our partner's body when we are in a relationship. We may be missing not just that other person but the stability and familiarity that their influence brought. They were influencing parts of us we may not even have noticed or known about. Studies show that our breathing

---

[53]Diamond, L. M., Hicks, A. M. and Otter-Henderson, K. D. 'Every time you go away: Changes in affect, behavior, and physiology associated with travel-related separations from romantic partners', *Journal of Personality and Social Psychology*, 95(2) (2008), 385–403. doi:10.1037/0022-3514.95.2.385

patterns,[54] our respiratory function,[55] our heart rate,[56] our sleep cycle[57] and even the level to which our body produces and regulates hormones like cortisol[58] and prolactin[59] can be influenced by the rhythms of our partner's body. Whatever our body did before that relationship can be significantly changed, and likewise it can be abruptly interrupted when that person is no longer around. For me, reading studies on this phenomenon felt unnerving and reassuring all at once. It was so strange to think that the way my heart pumped blood around my body, something so seemingly practical and physical, could be different when I was with someone I was emotionally connected to. No wonder we feel off-kilter when that person suddenly isn't there.

One of the most fascinating studies Sarah has sent me over the years was one carried out in Finland at the Aalto University School of Science and Technology in Espoo. In this study researchers monitored the heart rates of people

[54]Ferrer, E. and Helm, J. L. 'Dynamical systems modeling of physiological coregulation in dyadic interactions', *International Journal of Psychophysiology: Official Journal of the International Organization of Psychophysiology*, 88(3) (2013), 296–308. doi:10.1016/j.ijpsycho.2012.10.013

[55]Helm, J. L., Sbarra, D. A. and Ferrer, E. 'Coregulation of respiratory sinus arrhythmia in adult romantic partners', *Emotion*, 14(3) (2014), 522–31. doi:10.1037/a0035960

[56]Helm, J. L., Sbarra, D. and Ferrer, E. 'Assessing cross-partner associations in physiological responses via coupled oscillator models', *Emotion*, 12(4) (2012), 748–62. doi:10.1037/a0025036

[57]Yoon, H., Choi, S. H., Kim, S. K. et al. 'Human heart rhythms synchronize while co-sleeping', *Frontiers in Physiology*, 10 (2019), 190. doi:10.3389/fphys.2019.00190

[58]Saxbe, D. and Repetti, R. L. 'For better or worse? Coregulation of couples' cortisol levels and mood states', *Journal of Personality and Social Psychology*, 98(1) (2010), 92–103. doi:10.1037/a0016959

[59]Schneiderman, I., Kanat-Maymon, Y., Zagoory-Sharon, O. and Feldman, R. 'Mutual influences between partners' hormones shape conflict dialog and relationship duration at the initiation of romantic love', *Social Neuroscience*, 9(4) (2014), 337–51. doi:10.1080/17470919.2014.893925

taking part in a fire-walking experiment and of those who were observing them. The study found that all the participants in the fire-walking experience had a distinctive heart-rate 'signature', with a high peak distributed around the moment of the walk. As the researchers monitored those watching the experience, they found that the observers who were emotionally connected to those taking part (i.e. their family and friends) actually displayed the same heart-rate elevations to those doing the walk. Even though they were only watching the experience, their heart rates mirrored the activity of those of their loved ones. In addition to this, when the researchers looked at the heart rates of those observers who were not emotionally connected to the participants, incredibly, these did not change.[60] It was not the general excitement of fire-walking; it wasn't that everyone watching and taking part in the experiment was united in a similar physical response – it was only those observers with a close connection to the person doing the walk whose heart rates were affected. How wonderful to think that as we watch someone we love experience something, a part of our body can actually mirror theirs. How amazing that we can share something like a racing heartbeat just because we care about each other.

[60]Konvalinka, I., Xygalatas, D., Bulbulia, J., Schjødt, U., Jegindø, E.-M., Wallot, S., Van Orden, G. and Roepstorff, A. 'Synchronized arousal between performers and related spectators in a fire-walking ritual', *PNAS*, 108(20) (2011), 8514–9. doi:10.1073/pnas.1016955108

The flip side of all this, of course, is the impact of losing that connection. Just as there is a great deal of research around synchronicity and our ties to those we love, at the other end of the spectrum there is also research into how disruptive this loss can be. Not to be a huge downer, but the loss of this kind of bond can significantly throw us off balance, apparently to the degree that we can experience biobehavioural dysregulation, psychological disorganisation and even a full-blown stress response.[61] The research around this impact, though, is really all about the change, the shift from one status to another. We have been intertwined with someone else on a huge variety of levels, and so we need time to adjust and let our bodies settle into a new rhythm. If we consider the impact we are recovering from, perhaps we can be a little less terrified of how we currently feel. If our hearts, our breathing, our sleep and even the hormones floating around our bodies have been altered when we are with someone, perhaps we need to be realistic about how initially destabilising the loss of that influence can be. A bond has been altered and, according to the studies in this area, this really can change how we function at first.

---

[61]Sbarra, D. A. and Hazan, C. 'Coregulation, dysregulation, self-regulation: An integrative analysis and empirical agenda for understanding adult attachment, separation, loss, and recovery', *Personality and Social Psychology Review*, 12(2) (2008), 141–67. doi:10.1177/1088868308315702

So, how do we help ourselves acclimatise? How do we recover from this change? The previous rhythms and cycles within our bodies should naturally settle down as we are no longer romantically linked to that person, but we still have to recover from the impact of the loss. We also want to counteract the stress response that can come from this. We have already looked at ways of helping with the stress of shock and ways of releasing stress hormones like cortisol from our bodies, but here we are talking about the stress that can be induced specifically by the transition from being in a couple to suddenly being single and the strange gap this can leave. Separation and loneliness can trigger a stress response all of their own, along with feelings of isolation.

This is where, on repeat, I have read broadly the same advice. Yes, one bond has been broken and this break has been a kick in the head, but not all our bonds are broken – not all our relationships and not all our connections. While we try to recover from this change, we need to remember the bonds that we do have. We can still feel these connections; our hearts can still be tied to others, even if one particular heart is no longer around.

Helping Us Along the Way

Studies on the importance of social connections and community have shown that not only do we benefit from these interactions in many ways but we actually need them for our mental and physical health. There has been a great deal of research into this area over the past few decades and broadly, studies show that, to some degree, our health is tied to the strength of our social connections. Loneliness has been linked to increased risk of morbidity and mortality, while isolation has been found to activate a particular pattern of physiological and neural responses, which over time can mean poorer health and, again, an increased risk of mortality.[62] I don't think our biggest fear here should be that we are going to spontaneously drop dead from loneliness, but if research really does show a link between our health and social support that can even affect mortality, then increasing our social connections as much as possible can only be a positive thing. It is not only that social support correlates with a higher life expectancy[63] or that those people with strong social ties have shown increased resistance to disease and infections,[64] it is that having social support, or even

[62]Quadt, L., Esposito, G., Critchley, H. D. and Garfinkel, S. N. 'Brain-body interactions underlying the association of loneliness with mental and physical health', *Neuroscience and Biobehavioral Reviews*, 116 (2020), 283–300. doi:10.1016/j.neubiorev.2020.06.015

[63]Holt-Lunstad, J., Smith, T. B. and Layton, J. B. 'Social relationships and mortality risk: A meta-analytic review', *PLoS Medicine*, 7(7) (2010), e1000316. doi:10.1371/journal.pmed.1000316

[64]Uchino, B. N. 'Social support and health: A review of physiological processes potentially underlying links to disease outcomes', *Journal of Behavioral Medicine*, 29 (2006), 377–87. doi:10.1007/s10865-006-9056-5

just one supportive connection as opposed to none, can actually decrease your experience of pain, fear and stress. Yes, I'll be honest, initially these experiments started on rats, where rats in groups experienced less impact from electric shocks than those that were alone,[65] but these studies soon expanded to include humans too. The presence of a friend, for example, has been shown to decrease the impact of stress: studies looking at participants undergoing stress tests found that the subjects produced less cardiovascular activity and lower cortisol responses when they had a friend next to them.[66] A study at Yale University School of Nursing showed that 91% of pregnant women with high life stress and low social support had pregnancy-related complications, whereas only 33% of those with high life stress and high social support showed similar issues.[67] In several experiments looking at pain in relation to social support, participants reported feeling significantly less pain when viewing a photograph of a loved one than while undergoing the same level of pain without this image. Brain scans taken during the experiment even showed different readings when the participants perceived support (i.e. had their

[65]Davitz, J. R. and Mason, D. J. 'Socially facilitated reduction of a fear response in rats', *Journal of Comparative and Physiological Psychology*, 48(3) (1955), 149–51. doi:10.1037/h0046411

[66]Heinrichs, M., Baumgartner, T., Kirschbaum, C. and Ehlert, U. 'Social support and oxytocin interact to suppress cortisol and subjective responses to psychosocial stress', *Biological Psychiatry*, 54(12) (2003), 1389–98. doi:10.1016/s0006-3223(03)00465-7

[67]Nuckolls, K. B., Cassel, J. and Kaplan, B. H. 'Psychosocial assets, life crisis and the prognosis of pregnancy', *American Journal of Epidemiology*, 95(5) (1972), 431–41. doi:10.1093/oxfordjournals.aje.a121410

loved one's image with them) than when they did not, revealing decreased activity in neural regions that respond to threat and pain.[68]

So much of heartbreak is painful and stressful and frightening, so if we can alleviate this through keeping strong connections with those people we do have in our lives and utilising the incredible benefits of this support, then science (as well as, probably, our gut instinct) says to do so. It is more important than ever not to lock ourselves away. Not just because loneliness may be circling us right now, but because we really can be helped by the support of those around us as we try to recover from our heartbreak. We need to keep regular contact with those we love, and we need to increase time spent with supportive friends and family. If you are having a particularly bad heartbreak day, the stress and pain of this may be decreased by even just the presence of a good friend.

Battling loneliness is easier said than done. Who knows what your particular situation was before or is after this relationship, and so many of us are not just linked to our partners themselves but to the world that stretches beyond them, to their friends and family; even the places you went

[68]Eisenberger, N. I., Master, S. L., Inagaki, T. K., Taylor, S. E., Shirinyan, D., Lieberman, M. D. and Naliboff, B. D. 'Attachment figures activate a safety signal-related neural region and reduce pain experience', *PNAS*, 108(28) (2011), 11721–6. doi:10.1073/pnas.1108239108

together can become part of the loss. So here are some tips for trying to handle loneliness and some ways to keep our mental health as positive as possible. These are taken from a huge project run by the BBC in 2018 in partnership with the Wellcome Collection called the Loneliness Experiment, in which over 55,000 people took part, making it the largest survey of its kind to date. The data collected included useful coping techniques that these thousands of people actively used to counteract the negative effects of loneliness. These were collated into a podcast series, still available online, which outlines episode by episode the techniques found to be most effective.[69]

Number one on the list was distraction. This could involve the immediate distraction techniques we talked about earlier or longer-term goals such as hobbies, study or work. You don't have to already have a huge passion for something to throw yourself into a hobby; this could be a new thing you try while loneliness is a little more present – maybe a hobby you've never pursued but have always meant to. Something that can distract your mind from ruminating and getting stuck on feeling alone. Yes, maybe we didn't see all this coming, but who knows, maybe this is the year we take up knitting. Maybe

---

[69]BBC Radio 4. 'How You Can Feel Less Lonely' [podcast]. All in the Mind (2018). Available at: <https://www.bbc.co.uk/programmes/p06mp7zv>

something wonderful will come from throwing ourselves into an unfamiliar activity, and we will not only be able to use it for distraction but actually find something new to enjoy.

New social activities also ranked highly on the list of techniques, so even if, for example, you typically choose to exercise alone and enjoy running on a treadmill, maybe this is the time to try a social exercise class. If, like me, you know that you find zumba classes mortifying, just try to pick something from the huge list of possible classes and activities that are social on some level. You don't have to be chatting away to other people in this activity the entire time – even just being in a social setting where you are united in some way can lift your spirits a little. A book club, a yoga class… whatever feels like something you can try. You don't need to do this forever – this is just about taking a chance on something new and preventing too much time inside your own head.

The third technique that this project revealed (which is complemented by studies showing that reappraisal is an effective technique in combatting loneliness) is to 'reframe' our thinking about spending time alone. This technique is about adjusting our mindset and approaching time alone as a positive concept rather than a negative one. A recent study on college students struggling with loneliness showed that participants who read about the benefits of solitude experienced a smaller reduction in positive mood after being alone than those who did not. Just reading the text they were given on the positives of time alone, whether they actively tried to believe it or not, had an impact on how much time by themselves distressed them.[70]

Other methods found to be helpful by the thousands of people who took part in the Loneliness Experiment were: talking to friends and family about how they were feeling (i.e. admitting to being lonely rather than hiding it), starting a conversation with someone new and looking for the good in those around them. This last point is really to do with the isolating effects of loneliness and how, when we are isolated, we can become increasingly insular, our trust in others decreasing and our mammalian self-protection instincts shooting up. Isolation can have a kind of snowball effect where the more we are alone, the more we believe that external contact or influences are a possible threat. This is likely to manifest in very subtle ways for the average person spending a tad more time alone than usual, as opposed to someone in full-blown solitary confinement, but distrust

[70]Rodriguez, M., Bellet, B. W. and McNally, R. J. 'Reframing time spent alone: Reappraisal buffers the emotional effects of isolation', *Cognitive Therapy and Research*, 44 (2020), 1052–67. doi:10.1007/s10608-020-10128-x

of others can be a side effect. An eleven-year study at the University of Chicago found that it is possible to get stuck in a kind of loneliness loop, where loneliness can make us more self-centred, and then the more self-centred we become, the more lonely we get.[71] The Loneliness Experiment suggests that in trying actively to look for the good in others we can redress this balance.

If we can, where possible, use a variety of these techniques to counteract loneliness, we will find recovering from our broken hearts noticeably easier. There is little chance of not feeling lonely at all during this time, as this is such a common symptom of a break-up, but we can try to notice when that feeling is creeping in and use some of these methods to stop it taking over. I know phoning Sarah from the side of the road in the middle of New York kept me sane, even when I was freezing my bottom off and standing in two feet of snow. Talking about feeling lonely really helped, and as time passed I met more people, stopped getting lost and got really into pizza slices, to the degree that my roommate posted pizza back to me when I finally moved home to London. What an impression to leave on someone. If I had never leant on Sarah, though, and used social support to get me through that time, then maybe I would never have made

---

[71] University of Chicago. 'Loneliness contributes to self-centeredness for sake of self-preservation: Study finds positive feedback loop between behaviors', ScienceDaily (13 June 2017). Available at: <www.sciencedaily.com/releases/2017/06/170613102013.htm>

all the happy memories I did. We are social beings, and so during our heartbreak recovery we need more than ever to nurture our social connections. Even if it is difficult, even if our energy is depleted, we need to try our hardest to stay social and connected, as it may just help our broken hearts heal a little bit faster.

CHAPTER SIX

Recovering From the Recovery

I wish that, among all the reassurance, tips and insights I have found in the wonderful world of neuroscience, there were also a wonderful algorithm that would give us a date and time when this heartbreak would be over. So far, though, science keeps on telling me that although it may be clever, it is not yet magical. Some of us are recovering from a short, powerful romance, while others may have had a long and complex marriage. There is no one-size-fits-all answer to this process, and searching for that elusive concept of closure can be the hardest part of the whole thing. I think this is why professionals use the term 'acceptance' when they refer to grief rather than 'closure' – searching for closure is the kind of quest that can really drive us mad. I've lost many hours trying to make every little part of a relationship and break-up fit into one neat explanation, when really I just needed to find a way of accepting that it had happened at all.

Acceptance sounds so pleasant and calm, like it should be the easy bit of the process, the cup of mint tea at the end of the meal. In reality, there is a sort of blurry daze to the other end of the healing process, like waking up on a long-haul flight to a tray of indistinguishable breakfast foods. I know that even as I started to feel better there was a part of me that just wanted to go 'Huh? What just happened?!' There should be some sort of heartbreak spa facility just for those of us recovering from the recovery, giving us back our strength after all this healing.

The most encouraging study I found relating to acceptance involved, in a way, the simplest concept – simple and yet reassuringly validated by a little science. This study was conducted by the same clever team at the University of Missouri–St. Louis who used negative reappraisal and distraction techniques to positive effect, but this experiment tested the method of trying to 'own our feelings',[72] essentially suggesting that we give ourselves permission to feel the way we do. Recovery is not all about moving on but also about accepting these experiences and feelings as a part of our lives. We are allowed to have fallen in love, to have liked that person or embarked on that relationship. We didn't mess up or fail.

[72]Langeslag, S. J. E. and Sanchez, M. E. 'Down-regulation of love feelings after a romantic break-up: Self-report and electrophysiological data', *Journal of Experimental Psychology: General*, 147(5) (2018), 720–33. doi:10.1037/xge0000360

Even if we feel terrible in the period of heartbreak, we don't have to feel terrible about the relationship or about the feelings we have had. This study asked participants to reappraise their feelings around the relationship they were recovering from. This is a cognitive therapy employed within acceptance and commitment therapy (ACT) and can be used in various moments when we experience negative emotions. For example, if we hear back about a job application and we didn't get the role, using this approach we would tell ourselves that it is OK to feel sad and to experience that sadness without judgement. This technique is all about accepting our feelings rather than trying to conquer them. In this experiment participants were given simple statements that allowed the reader to accept whatever loving feelings they experienced rather than seeing these as mistakes. These statements were as broad as 'It's OK to love someone you're no longer with' or 'Love is part of life', with the participants all asked to concentrate on them for a few seconds while they were shown on a screen. Incredibly, concentrating on these relatively generic statements actually made a difference to how the participants felt about their ex-partners. It wasn't that they were no longer sad or heartbroken, but they were less captivated by the heartbreakers themselves. This was evaluated by taking LLP (late positive potentials) readings, which is a way of recording how much motivated attention someone gives another person or object. When the men and women taking part in the experiment used the method of accepting their feelings, their LLP figures decreased. They were less affected by the images of their ex-partners and gave them less focus and attention. If we are trying to let that person go and no longer be thrown by the idea of them or their existence, then this is quite encouraging. The sentences were not specifically tailored to each person's experience or relationship – they just gave people permission to let go of any judgement of their own feelings.

Acceptance sounds a little abstract sometimes – like, even if I decide I want to accept all this, how do I do it? What is my method? Do I just tell myself I accept it and hope acceptance kicks in? Well, in a way, that is what we can do. It's not a waste of time to try allowing ourselves to accept how we feel and to remind ourselves that whatever we feel is permitted. For me, this concept felt quite freeing. Simple, yes, but encouraging. It was uplifting to hear that people who spent a few minutes concentrating on the idea of acceptance and giving themselves a little judgement-free breathing space were less transfixed by the person they were trying to separate themselves from than before. Perhaps when looking for that elusive closure we all want to find, we can nudge the process along a little by practicing less self-judgement and a little more self-approval.

Many of the techniques I've read about when delving into the world of neuroscience have been subtle, gentle changes to our normal routine. Something like going for a walk in nature or even just changing your usual route to include more trees doesn't sound that groundbreaking. I'm not sure I would even have trusted theories like these if they hadn't come via science and studies. There is so much advice out there, so many things we could do with our time, that just knowing something had been investigated thoroughly and had yielded positive results gave me more reassurance that it might work for me. It was a happy accident that Sarah and I became friends and that the person whose shoulder I would cry on whenever a boy didn't call was also someone so full of facts and figures. She is someone whose mind naturally works analytically, and by fortunate chance her approach appeases the suspicious, cynical part of me that always wants to know *why* I should get more sleep or *why* I should distract myself from thoughts of that handsome bartender.

Perhaps you are more open and trusting than me and don't need the data to reassure you, but the more studies I have read, the calmer I have felt. To read about the post-break-up brain and know that love withdrawal is a real thing? That we're essentially addicts trying to recover? Those studies probably gave me more relief than any other resources I have come across. I think when we are rejected we see ourselves through the eyes of the person who rejected us, and it is hard not to be very self-critical. But when you see study after study looking at group after group of broken-hearted people, all going through similar experiences, it can be a reminder that this happens to nearly everyone. Many people have been heartbroken before us and many people will be heartbroken afterwards. We are loving, feeling beings and the stinger that comes along with that is our ability to feel pain and loss.

The wonderful thing about looking at something as emotional as heartbreak through the lens of neuroscience is that it can give us an anchor to hold on to. I hope you will find the same reassurance and encouragement from all these interesting studies as I have, and that some of the techniques which have been shown to help others – such as spending time in nature, physical exercise, turning to your support network or simply crying it all out – help you too. Although we are all going to get through this in different ways, having a good selection of techniques to choose from will hopefully help us to figure out our own personal strategy. It may sound cheesy, but it is true that time is a great healer, so if we do what we can to ease this transition then our hearts will eventually mend. We will not be broken-hearted forever; we will go out into the world and date again, telling ever-so-slightly rehearsed anecdotes with the best of them.

Good luck, friend. I'm rooting for you.

Acknowledgements

Thank you to my wonderful friend Professor Sarah Garfinkel, who is not only a brilliant scientist but a kind, supportive soul. Thank you also to everyone at Fairlight Books, especially Louise Boland and my editor Laura Shanahan.

About the Author

Ziella Bryars is a writer and producer. She founded the new writing theatre show *Love Bites* in 2008. Her plays include *Blind Date*, *True Love*, *A Room on Greek Street* and *Down in One*. Her work has been performed at Southwark Playhouse, the Live Theatre Newcastle and the Red Room New York, as well as the various London venues to host Love Bites over the years. Her love of romantic comedies and the chaos of modern dating have led Ziella to write extensively about love and relationships. She is currently working on her first novel and a limited television series. She lives in London.

LUCINDA FORD

How to Sleep

Introducing eight easy-to-use techniques for
falling asleep, *How to Sleep: A Natural Method* is
an indispensable companion for those who find it
difficult to fall asleep and stay asleep.

When sleeplessness becomes a regular occurrence,
it can set up a vicious cycle of fatigue, anxiety and
sleepless nights. Finding ways to turn off the racing
mind and negative thoughts or stress when going
to sleep is an essential step, allowing you to break
that vicious cycle and move towards a place of better
well-being. The eight simple sleep techniques, along
with their accompanying notes, are designed to calm
the mind and allow sleep to come naturally. They are
distilled from the best of thinking from the East and
the West, including cognitive behavioural therapy,
mindfulness and meditation, taking lessons from each
of these methods on how best to quiet your mind and
find a calm place from which to fall asleep.

'How to Sleep *gives valuable advice and tips to*
help with many of the leading causes of sleeplessness
without people needing a PhD to understand it.'
— Ian Stockbridge, MNCS (Accred.),
MBABCP, MBACP

LYNN MORRISON

How to Market Your Book

These days, regardless of whether a book is self-published or traditionally published, there will be an expectation on the author to take an active role in marketing their book. Based on a series of interviews with successful authors from both sides of the publishing divide and both sides of the pond, Lynn lays out in detail the marketing strategies that have worked for them, alongside an explanation of how book marketing works based on her own long-standing career as a senior marketing exec.

From developing social media tactics and arranging promotional events to handling press and trying to start viral campaigns, Lynn offers practical advice designed to help an author find a book marketing strategy that best works for them, based on their personal strengths and budget.

'Morrison turns the overwhelming task of marketing into bite-size tips and tutorials that anyone can implement.'
— Stephanie Jankowski, author of *Schooled*

LYNN MORRISON

How to Be Published

Theoretically there has never been a better time to become a published writer. But for anyone looking to venture into today's publishing landscape, it can be a daunting prospect – self-publish? Look for an agent? Go direct to an indie publisher? And what exactly is digital-first publishing?

How to Be Published is the first book to offer an unbiased guide to the pros and cons of self-publishing versus traditional publishing, along with all the myriad options in between – helping an author navigate the complex world of publishing and find the best path for them, their book and their writing aspirations.

'Navigating the murky waters of first-time publishing can be intimidating. I wish I'd had a guide like this when I was first deciding between traditional and self-publishing.'
— Mary Widdicks, author of the *Mermaid Asylum* series